NURSING MNEMONICS:
EASIEST WAY TO REMEMBER

Introduction

If you want a way to remember anything, from names of people to important dates, the mnemonic techniques are a brilliant way to help. They are also used in mentalism for various purposes.

What is Mnemonics?

Mnemonics come from the ancient Greek word 'mnemothia,' which means 'to remember.'

It is a technique that involves a system in which you link new information to pre-existing information. It is a powerful tool that all of us use daily, without even realizing it.

The term 'mnemonic' often refers to a 'memory aid.' For example, when trying to remember something like the colors of the rainbow or the order in which you need to pick up your dry cleaning, we use mnemonics. They can also be used for remembering things like birthdays and anniversaries or other special occasions.

History

The term 'mnemonics' has been around for a long time. It is believed that the first mnemonic was developed by a Greek philosopher named Aristotle in his book called 'Metaphysics.' If you analyze the title of his book, you'll notice it contains many mnemonic words; such as 'matter,' 'motion,' and 'virtue.' Aristotle chose these words to represent the three types of memory we have - visual, verbal, and auditory.

In the 1700s, a German scientist named Korzybski was working on theories about how humans process language. He suggested that several specific words/phrases could be used to facilitate human learning and retention.

Some of the most famous mnemonic devices were developed in the 1800s, including the one used for remembering the order of colors in a rainbow (ROY G BIV). It is said that they were developed by an English professor called Richard Grey.

Many people still use them today without even realizing that they are using mnemonics.

How Mnemonics Work

The classical mnemonic system includes:

- **Encoding**

This is where you link new information to old information that is already in your memory. Therefore, you begin to associate the new information with the old information.

- Decoding

This is where you try and use your memory to generate the perceptual images you made during encoding. This is how you imagine yourself riding a bike, and then the bike has a different handlebar position. In studies about memory, it was found that these perceptual images which develop during encoding can be used to link together new information with old information.

The Representational System:

Why does this matter? As I like to explain things, it matters because now you may remember how to ride a bike next year. All you need to do is think of the perceptual images from when you first learned how to ride a bike, which means that you may be able to get access to the memory of how to ride a bike even if your long-term memory has been corrupted. After all, if you're not in a coma right now, you might be able to get access to your long-term memory. You only have a few seconds to try and remember how to ride a bike, but there's no point in doing this when your long-term memory is damaged anyway because that has no bearing on how you came to learn it. Your long-term memory is probably pretty bad already. It's just not terminal enough yet for you to notice it. But wait! The effect doesn't stop there. You may want to try and remember how to ride a bike next year, or ever. The mnemonic system will help you in that regard by allowing you to make perceptual images of the same things repeatedly.

How Mnemonics are Used in Mentalism

One of the most famous mnemonic techniques is called 'COLOR-AID.' It involves using various colors -green, blue, orange, red, etc. In this example, I'll be using Red:

1. When you need to remember information about a person
2. You think of an image related to that person
3. You then associate red with the person's name
4. This is the image you will require to use when you need to remember the information
5. The information about a person can be linked to the name due to this mnemonic system of using perceptual images

Chapter 1: Cardiovascular Mnemonics

Adrenergic Receptors

Beta-1 affects the heart (1 Heart)

Beta-2 affects the Lungs (2 Lungs)

Beta-1 and beta-2 are adrenergic receptors. There are also alpha-1, alpha-2, and beta-3. Learn those also, but the two most common you'll see in nursing school will likely be beta-1 and beta-2. Beta-1 receptors primarily affect the heart. For example, beta-1 agonists help to increase cardiac output and heart rate. Beta-2 receptors primarily affect the lungs. For example, beta-2 agonists help to relax the smooth muscle in the lungs, causing bronchial dilation. These are mostly used in the treatment of asthma.

Cardiac Conduction – Electrical Pathway

On Saturdays, I Avoid Bee Hives with Bumble Bees in the Park Forest

SA Node – AV Node – Bundle of HIS – Bundle Branches (right and left) – Purkinje's Fibers

When I was in school, I had a heck of a time remembering two things: the blood flow through the heart and the conduction pathway through the heart. This mnemonic isn't ideal, but it helped me recall it in a pinch. The first signal comes from the sinoatrial (SA) node and proceeds to the atrioventricular (AV) node. From here, the signal goes to the Bundle of HIS and then to the right and left bundle branches. Finally, the electrical current gets to the Purkinje's Fibers.

Cardiac Tamponade – Symptoms

"Beck's Triad" in 3D

- Distant heart sounds
- Decreased arterial BP
- Distended jugular veins

Alternative...

Have More Juice

- Hypotension
- Muffled heart sounds
- JVD (Jugular vein distention)

Cardiac tamponade is when there is so much f fluid around the heart that it causes compression, decreasing the strength at which the heart can work. Common signs and symptoms include distant heart sounds, hypotension, and distended jugular veins. Together, these encompass what's referred to as Beck's Triad. Follow one or both of these mnemonics to help you remember.

Cardiogenic Shock – Source

RIP

- Rhythm
- Ischemia
- Pump

Cardiogenic shock happens when there isn't enough blood flow in the body due to heart failure. This could be because of the heart rhythm, ischemia, and pump problems. If the heart is in a rhythm that can't maintain perfusion, it could lead to cardiogenic shock (supraventricular tachycardia, atrial fibrillation, etc.). If there is a lack of blood flow getting to the heart, such as in myocardial ischemia, it could also cause this problem. The heart muscle can get weaker, making it less effective. This is the most common reason. The last cause of cardiogenic shock in this mnemonic, "pump," is when the heart isn't pumping properly because of a mechanical issue like endocarditis, valve disorders, or cardiomyopathies.

Cardiogenic Shock – Treatment

HABIT

- Hydrate
- Antiarrhythmics
- Balloon pump (intra-aortic)
- Inotropes
- Treat symptoms

Cardiogenic shock happens when there isn't enough blood flow in the body due to heart failure. Treatment goals will be to increase the heart's strength and ability to pump. Depending on the underlying problem, the patient will need to be given fluids, antiarrhythmics, inotropes, and even an intra-aortic balloon pump if necessary. As with anything else, treat the symptoms as they arise.

Circulation Through the Heart

Heart Valves in Order

Toilet Paper My Ass

- Tricuspid
- Pulmonary
- Mitral
- Aortic

Circulation through the heart is tricky to learn. I know that the mnemonic on the top is very difficult and may not help at all. This is a topic that may just require straight memorization. But I thought I'd give it a shot anyway. The bottom mnemonic for the heart valves is maybe a little more helpful.

CHF (Congestive Heart Failure) – Treatment

UNLOAD FAST

- Upright position
- Nitrates
- Lasix
- Oxygen
- ACE Inhibitors
- Digoxin
- Fluid restriction
- Afterload reduction
- Sodium restriction
- Tests (digoxin level, ABGs, BNP)

For a patient with CHF, you are going to want to "UNLOAD" the extra fluid "FAST." Keep these patients in the upright position to help facilitate breathing and make them more comfortable. Nitrates may be ordered to help decrease demand on the heart. They may need oxygen to help ventilation, but also to get more oxygen to the heart. In order to reduce the fluid, diuretics such as Lasix can be given. These patients should also be put on fluid restrictions and a low sodium diet. Water follows sodium, so the more salt in their diet, the more water will hang around. ACE inhibitors can be used to treat hypertension, something common in this patient population. Digoxin can help to improve the strength of each heart contraction and aid in circulation. These patients should have regular labs done, such as ABGs and BNP levels. If they are on digoxin, they will need to have digoxin levels checked.

EKG Basics

PAC the things from QVC TV Rapidly

- P wave: Atrial Contraction (depolarization)
- QRS: Ventricular Contraction (depolarization)
- T wave: Ventricular Repolarization

This one is tough, but so many people have a hard time remembering what they're looking at when they look at an EKG. Some mnemonic had to be considered. Good luck—I hope you can think of a better one. The way I remember it is by using the phrase "Pack the things from QVC TV Rapidly." In case you weren't aware, QVC is a program on TV where you can call in or go online to buy things while they are on sale for a short period of time. So, come with me on this silly mnemonic journey.

After you buy them, you want to PACK them up. The P wave on an EKG represents depolarization or Atrial Contraction.

You bought the things from QVC. The QRS complex on an EKG represents a continuing part of depolarization or Ventricular Contraction.

You didn't just buy the things from QVC—you bought them on TV Rapidly. The T wave on an EKG represents Ventricular Repolarization.

EKG Lead Placement

For a standard five lead EKG, follow these simple rules to remember where they go on the chest.

1. Smoke over Fire (Black over Red)
2. White on Right
3. Green: Gallbladder
4. Brown "Around" the Sternum

As easy as this sounds, a basic 5-lead EKG lead placement still gets misplaced by even the most seasoned nurses. But it's so simple if you can remember this mnemonic. Start with the left side: smoke over a fire. Think of the black lead as the smoke and place it in the upper left half of the body (usually near the left shoulder/chest). The red lead (fire) should then be placed under the black lead on the lower half of the body (typically on the lower left abdomen or ribcage). Once you have these two, move on to the next part of the mnemonic.

The white lead placement should be easy to remember because it rhymes with the right, which is where it needs to be. This is typically placed opposite of the black lead and is usually around the right shoulder/chest area. The green lead is the one and only lead that starts with 'G,' just like the word, 'gallbladder,' This lead should be on the lower right side of the body and is usually placed in the general area of the gallbladder (in the lower right abdomen or ribcage). Finally, the brown lead should be placed 'around' the Sternum (brown: around). For the basic five lead-ins V1 position, this is just to the right of mid-sternum.

Heart Blocks

Popular poem to help remember the different types of heart block

- 1st Degree: If R is far from P, we call that a 1st degree
- 2nd Degree, Type 1 (Wenkebach): Longer, longer, longer, drop. Now we have a Wenkebach
- 2nd Degree, Type 2 (Mobitz II): If some P's just can't get through, now we have a Mobitz II
- 3rd Degree (Complete Heart Block): If the P's and Q's cannot agree, now we have a 3rd degree

1st-degree heart block is characterized by a P-R interval greater than 0.2 seconds. It looks like a typical sinus rhythm, but the p wave is farther from the r wave than normal.

2nd degree, type 1 heart block is also known as a Wenkebach. You may see or hear either term. In this type of block, the p wave goes further away from the r wave with each beat. Eventually, a beat is skipped, and the cycle starts over.

2nd degree, type II heart block is also known as a Mobitz II. In this type of block, the rhythm appears normal until a complex suddenly gets dropped without warning. The P-R interval is constant, and it just looks like a beat gets skipped.

3rd-degree heart block, also known as complete heart block, is where the P waves and the QRS complex don't communicate with each other at all. There is no reason where a P wave or a QRS will show up.

Heart Failure – Left Sided

POACHED

- Pulmonary congestion
- Orthopnea
- Adventitious breath sounds
- Cough
- Hemoptysis
- Extreme weakness
- Dyspnea

Alternative…

SCORED

- Sleepy (fatigue)
- Cyanosis/Confusion
- Orthopnea
- Rales/Restlessness
- Extreme weakness
- Dyspnea

Left-sided heart failure happens when the left ventricle isn't pumping effectively enough. Since it's not getting blood out of the heart in sufficient volumes, fluid builds up into the lungs, causing pulmonary edema. These patients will have difficulty breathing and will be very weak. They might have a cough, and sometimes you see hemoptysis (frothy pink sputum is a hallmark symptom). The lungs will sound wet in the form of rales or crackles.

Heart Failure – Right Sided

BOUNCED

- Bloating
- Oliguria
- Unable to eat
- Nausea

- Cyanosis/Cool legs
- Edema
- Distended neck veins (JVD)

Alternative…

WARHEAD

- Weight gain (because of retained fluid)
- Anorexia
- Reduced urine output
- Hepatomegaly
- Edema
- Ascites
- Distended neck veins (JVD)

Right-sided heart failure usually happens when fluid in the lungs causes the right ventricle to work harder and eventually pump less effectively. Although some other factors could be in play, it is usually left-sided heart failure that causes it. It's like a vicious cycle. The left ventricle can't clear fluid from the lungs, and the right ventricle has a difficult time pumping against that extra fluid. When the right ventricle fails, fluid will start to back up to the rest of the body. Common symptoms include generalized edema, ascites, jugular venous distention, enlarged liver, decreased urine output, loss of appetite, nausea, and weight gain (due to the retained fluid).

Chapter 2: Pharmacy Mnemonics

Amiodarone: action, side effects

6 P's

- Prolongs action potential duration
- Photosensitivity
- Pigmentation of skin
- Peripheral neuropathy
- Pulmonary alveolitis and fibrosis
- Peripheral conversion of T4 to T3 inhibited

Antiarrhythmics: Class 1

Double Quarter Pounder with Lettuce, Mayo & Tomato, and More Fries Please!

Class I-A

- D - Disopyramide
- Q - Quinidine
- P - Procainamide

Class I-b

- L - Lidocaine
- M - Mexeletine
- T - Tocainide

Class I- C

- M - Moricizine
- F - Flecainide
- P - Propefanone

Antibiotics

MEDICATE

- M - Monitor superinfections
- E - Evaluate renal / liver functions
- D - Diarrhea – take yogurt
- I - Inform provider before taking other meds

- C - Cultures before initial dose
- A - Alcohol is out, ask about allergy
- T - Take the full course (of pills)
- E - Evaluate cultures, WBC, temperature, blood

Anticancer drugs: undesirable effects

BARFS

- B - Bone marrow depression
- A - Alopecia
- R - Retching – nausea / vomiting
- F - Fear and anxiety
- S - Stomatitis

Antihypertensive drugs: ACE inhibitors (ends in -pril)

Tom Eats Large Pizzas and Runs Fast In Benz Car

- T - Trandolapril
- E - Enapril
- L - Lisinopril
- P - Perindopril
- A - Ramipril
- R - Fosinopril
- F - Fosinopril
- I - Imidapril
- B - Benazepril
- C - Captopril

Antihypertensive drugs: Beta-blockers (ends in -lol)

PACEMAN BB

- P - Propanolol
- A - Atenolol
- C - Celiprolol
- E - Esmolol
- M - Metopolol
- A - Acebutolol
- N - Nevibulol
- B - Betazolol
- B - Bisoprolol

Antihypertensive drugs: Calcium antagonists

VINDANF

- V - Verapamil
- I - Isradipine
- N - Nifedipine
- D - Diltiazem
- A - Amlodipine
- N - Nicardipine
- F - Felodipine

Aspirin: side effects

ASPIRIN

- A - Asthma
- S - Salicyalism
- P - Peptic ulcer disease / Phosphorylation-oxidation uncoupling / PPH / Platelet disaggregation / Premature closure of PDA
- I - Intestinal blood loss
- R - Reye's syndrome
- I - Idiosyncrasy
- N - Noise (tinnitus)

Atropine use: tachycardia or bradycardia:

A goes with B

- Atropine used clinically to treat Bradycardia

Beta-blockers: cardioselectivity beta-blockers

Beta-blockers Acting Exclusively at Myocardium.

- B - Betaxolol
- A - Acebutelol
- E - Esmolol
- A - Atenolol
- M - Metoprolol

Birth Control Pills: Complications

ACHES

- A - Abdominal pain
- C - Chest pain
- H - Headaches
- E - Eye problems
- S - Severe leg pain

Bradycardia: Drugs

IDEA

- I - Isoproterenol
- D - Dopamine
- E - Epinephrine
- A - Atropine

Calcium channel blocker: Its uses

CHASM

- C - Cerebral Vasospasm / CHF
- H - Hypertension
- A - Angina
- S - Supraventricular tachyarrhythmia
- M - Migraines

Captopril (ACE inhibitor): Side Effects

CAPTOPRIL

- C - Cough
- A - Angioedema / Agranulocystosis
- P - Protenuria / Potassium excess
- T - Taste changes
- O - Orthostatis hypotension
- P - Pregnancy contraindications / Pancreatitis / Pressure drops
- R - Renal failure / Rash
- I - Indomethacin inhibition
- L - Leukopenia / Liver toxicity

Corticosteroids: Side Effects

CUSHINGS BAD MD

- C - Cataracts
- U - Up all night (sleep disturbances)
- S - Suppression of the HPA axis
- H - Hypertension
- I - Infections
- N - Necrosis (avascular)
- G - Gain Weight
- S - Striae

- B - Bone loss (osteoporosis)
- A - Acne
- D - Diabetes

- M - Myopathy
- D - Depression and emotional changes

Corticosteroid: side effects

CUSHINGOID MAP

- C - Cataracts
- U - Ulcers
- S - Skin: striae, thinning, bruising
- H - Hypertension/ Hirsutism / Hyperglycemia
- I - Infections
- N - Necrosis, avascular necrosis of the femoral head
- G - Glycosuria
- O - Osteoporosis, obesity
- I - Immunosuppression
- D - Diabetes mellitus

- M - Myopathy
- A - Adipose tissue hypertrophy
- P - Pancreatitis

Corticosteroid: Side Effects

STEROID May Cause CUSHING

- S - Skin thinning, Striae
- T - Teratogenicity
- E - Euphoria
- R - Retardation of growth
- O - Obesity, Osteoporosis
- I - Infection
- D - Diabetes

- M - Muscle weakness

- C - Cataract

- C - Cushing habitus
- U - Ulceration
- S - Suppression of the HPA axis
- H - Healing delay
- I - Immunosuppression
- N - Necrosis of head femur
- G - Glaucoma

Emergency drugs LEAN on

- L - Lidocaine
- E - Epinephrine
- A - Atropine
- N - Narcan

Folate deficiency: Causes

A FOLIC DROP

- A - Alcoholism

- F - Folic acid antagonists
- O - Oral contraceptives
- L - Low dietary intake
- I - Infection with Giardia
- C - Celia sprue

- D - Dilantin
- R - Relative folate deficiency
- O - Old
- P - Pregnancy

Gynecomastia causing drugs

DISCOS

- D - Digoxin
- I - Isoniazid
- S - Spironolactone
- C - Cimetidine
- O - Oestrogens
- S - Stilboestrol

Hypertension treatment ABCD

- A - ACE inhibitors / Angil antagonists
- B - Beta blockers
- C - Calcium antagonists
- D - Diuretics

Hypervitaminosis A: signs and symptoms

HARD

- H - Headache/ Hepatomegaly
- A - Anorexia/ Alopecia
- R - Really painful bones
- D - Dry skin/ Drowsiness

Ipecac: contraindications

4 Cs

- C - Comatose
- C - Convulsing
- C - Corrosive
- C - hydroCarbon

Lidocaine (antiarrhythmic): characteristics

LIDOCAINE

- L - Local anesthetic
- I - ICU popular antiarrhythmic
- D - Digitalis toxicity
- O - Orally inactive
- C - Cimetidine + Propanolol
- A - Automaticity reduction
- I - Inactive sodium channels
- N - Nystagmus
- E - ECG changes / Eye effects

Medication administration checklist

TRAMP

- T - Time Check the chart for the last time that the medication was given.
- R - Route Oral, IV, etc.
- A - Amount (dose). Check the chart for the dosing information.
- M - Medication. Verify the correct medication. Be aware of look-alike and sound-alike names.
- P – Patient. Ask the patient's name and check their ID band to verify.

Methotrexate: adverse effects

BHARAT

- B - Bone marrow suppression
- H - Hepatotoxicity
- A - Alopecia
- R - renal diseases
- A - Abdominal symptoms
- T - Teratogenicity

Methyldopa: side effects

METHYLDOPA

- M - Mental retardation
- E - Electrolyte impalance
- T - Tolerance

- H - Headache / Hypatotoxicity
- Y - psychological upset
- L - Lactation in female
- D - Dry mouth
- O - Oedema
- P - Parkinsonism
- A - Anemia

Morphine: side effects

MORPHINE

- M   Myosis
- Out of it (sedation)
- R   Respiratory depression
- P   Pneumonia (aspiration)
- H   Hypotension
- I   Infrequency (constipation, urinary retention)
- N   Nausea
- E   Emesis

Niacin

NIACIN

- N - Note liver function tests – regular intervals
- I - Itching and flushing
- A - Aspirin before Niacin may decrease
- C - Contraindications: hepatic disease, pregnancy
- I - Instruct to take with food and at bedtime
- N - No high cholesterol foods

Parkinson's: medications

Ali Loves Boxing Matches

- A - Amantadine (Symmetrel)
- L - Levodopa
- B - Bromocriptine (Parlodel)
- M - Mao-Inhibitors

Photosensitivity-causing drugs

PQRST

- P - Phenothiazine, Psoralen
- Q - Quinines
- R - Retinoids
- S - Suphonamides
- T - Tetracyclines, Thiazines

Respiratory depression: inducing drugs

STOP breathing

- S - Sedatives and hypnotics
- T - Trimethoprim
- O - Opiates
- P - Polymyxins

Selective serotonin reuptake

- inhibitor (SSRI): Adverse effects 3 Ss

    - S - Stomach upset
    - S - Sexual dysfunction
    - S - Serotonin syndrome

- **SSRI (Selective Seratonin Reuptake Inhibitor: drugs**

Effective For Sadness, Panic, and Compulsions

    - E - Escitalopram
    - F - Fluoxetine, Fluvoxamine
    - S - Sertroline
    - P - Paroxetine
    - C - Citalopram

Steroids: side effects

BECLOMETHASONE

- B - Buffalo hump
- E - Easy bruising

- C - Cataracts
- L - Larger appetite
- O - Obesity
- M - Moonface
- E - Euphoria
- T - Thin arms and legs
- H - Hypertension / hyperglycaemia
- A - Avascular necrosis of femoral head
- S - Skin thinning
- O - Osteoporosis
- N - Negative nitrogen balance
- E - Emotional liability

Steroids: side effects

5 Ss

- S - Sick (easier to get sick)
- S - Sad (causes depression)
- S - Sex (decreases libido)
- S - Salt (retains more, causes weight gain)
- S - Sugar (raises blood sugar)

Tuberculosis: drugs

RIPES

- R - Rifampicin
- I - Isoniazid
- P - Pyrazinamide
- E - Ethambutol
- S - Streptomycin

Vitamins: which is fat-soluble

KADE

- K - Vitamin K
- A - Vitamin A
- D - Vitamin D
- E - Vitamin E

Xylocaine: where not to use with epinephrine

Digital PEN

- D - Digits
- P - Penis
- E - Ear
- N - Nose

The vasoconstrictive effects of xylocaine with epinephrine help provide hemostasis while suturing. However, they may also cause local ischemic necrosis in digital structures such as the digits, tip of the nose, penis, ears, etc.

Drug Administration

DR. TIMED

- D - Dose
- R - Route

- T - Time
- I - Individual
- M - Medication
- E - Expiration date / Effect
- D - Documentation

Drugs deliverable by endotracheal tube

O NAVEL

- O - Oxygen

- N - Naloxone
- A - Atropine
- V - Ventolin (albuterol)
- E - Epinephrine
- L - Lidocaine

If you can't get IV access established and have the necessity to administer resuscitative meds, remember you have the airway and can give the above drugs. Drug delivery is enhanced if diluted with 10cc NS and rapidly introduced for aerosolization. Alternatively, the bare-bones version is ALE

Drug Interactions

These Drugs Can Interact

- T - Theophylline
- D - Dilantin
- C - Coumadin
- I - Ilosone

Drug-drug interactions

THE MAD WAR

- T - Tricyclic antidepressants
- H - Histamine antagonist
- E - Ethanol, Erythromycin
- M - MAO inhibitors
- A - Aminophylline, Aspirin
- D - Digoxin, Dilantin, Diuretics
- W - Warfarin
- A - Azole (antifungal), Antacids
- R - Rifampin

Chapter 3: Internal Medicine Mnemonics

ACEI: contraindictions

PARK:

- Pregnancy
- Allergy
- Renal artery stenosis
- K increase (hyperkalemia)

Anion gap metabolic acidosis: causes

A MUDPILE CAT:

- Alcohol
- Methanol
- Uremia
- Diabetic ketoacidosis
- Paraldehyde
- Iron/ Isoniazid
- Lactic acidosis
- Ethylene glycol
- Carbamazepine
- Aspirin
- Toluene

Hematology: key numbers

3 and 4 are key in in hematology:

1.34 cm 3 of oxygen is carried by a 1g. of hemoglobin. There is 3.4mg of iron in every gram of hemoglobin. There is a of 3.4 lobes per neutrophil. There is 34mg bilirubin from each gram of hemoglobin.

Macrocytic anemia: causes

ABCDEF:

- Alcohol + liver disease
- B12 deficiency
- Compensatory reticulocytosis (blood loss and hemolysis)

- Drug (cytotoxic and AZT)/ Dysplasia (marrow problems)
- Endocrine (hypothyroidism)
- Folate deficiency/ Fetus (pregnancy)

Metabolic acidosis: causes

KUSSMAL:

- Ketoacidosis
- Uraemia
- Sepsis
- Salicylates
- Methanol
- Alcohol
- Lactic acidosis

Non-gap acidosis: causes

HARD UP:

- Hyperalimentation
- Acetazolamide (carbonic anhydrase inhibitors)
- RTA
- Diarrhea
- Ureterosigmoidostomy
- Pancreatic fistula

Raynaud's disease: causes

BAD CT:

- Blood disorders (e.g., polycythaemia)
- Arterial (e.g., atherosclerosis, Buerger's)
- Drugs (e.g., beta-blockers)
- Connective tissue disorders (rheumatoid arthritis, SLE)
- Traumatic (e.g., vibration injury)

Ulcers: types

VAN:

- Venous/ Vasculitic
- Arterial

- Neuropathic

Acromegaly symptoms

ABCDEF:

- Arthralgia/ Arthritis
- Blood pressure raised
- Carpal tunnel syndrome
- Diabetes
- Enlarge med organs
- Field defect

Gynecomastia: common causes

GYNECOMASTIA:

- Genetic Gender disorder (Klinefelter)
- Young boy (pubertal)*
- Neonate*
- Estrogen
- Cirrhosis/ Cimetidine/ Ca Channel blockers
- Old age*
- Marijuana
- Alcoholism
- Spironolactone
- Tumors (Testicular & adrenal)
- Isoniazid/ Inhibition of testosterone
- Antineoplastics (Alkylating Agents)/ Antifungal(ketoconazole)

* Asterisk indicates physiologic cause.

Hypercalcemia causes

MD PIMPS ME:

- Malignancy
- Diuretics (thiazide the main culprit)
- Parathyroid (hyperparathyroidism)
- Immobilization/ Idiopathic
- Megadose of vitamins A, D
- Paget's disease
- Sarcoidosis

- Milk alkali syndrome
- Endocrine (Addison's disease, thyrotoxicosis)

Hypercalcemia: causes

GRIM FED:

- Granulomas (sarcoid, TB),
- Renal failure
- Immobility (esp. long term)
- Malignancy
- Familial (e.g., familial hypocalciuric hypercalcemia)
- Endocrine (see below for subtypes)
- Drugs (esp. thiazide diuretics, lithium)

Endocrine causes

PATH:

- Phaeochromocytoma
- Addison's disease
- Thyrotoxicosis
- Hyperparathyroidism

Hypercalcemia: differential

VITAMIN TRAPS:

- Vitamin A and D intoxication
- Immobilization
- Thyrotoxicosis
- Addison's disease/ Acidosis
- Milk-alkali syndrome
- Inflammatory disorders
- Neoplastic disease
- Thiazides, other drugs
- Rhabdomyolysis
- AIDS
- Paget's disease/ Parenteral nutrition/ Parathyroid disease
- Sarcoidosis

Pressure Sore: Norton Score

MAGIC:

- Mobility
- ADL
- General condition
- Incontinence
- Conscious level

Pruritus without rash: DDx

ITCHING DX:

- Infections (scabies, toxocariasis, etc.)
- Thyroidal and other endocrinopathies (e.g., diabetes mellitus)
- Cancer
- Hematologic diseases (e.g., iron deficiency)/ Hepatopathies/ HIV
- Idiopathic
- Neurotic
- Gravid (pruritus of pregnancy)
- Drugs
- eXcretory dysfunctions (e.g., uremia)

Rashes: The moment of appearance after fever

"RSCMTNE": Number of days after fever onset that a rash will appear:

- 1st Day: Rubella
- 2nd Days: Scarlet fever/ Smallpox
- 3rd Days: Chickenpox
- 4th Days: Measles (and see the Koplik spots one day prior to rash)
- 5th Days: Typhus & rickettsia (this is variable)
- 6th Days: Nothing
- 7th Days: Enteric fever (salmonella)

Alkalosis: metabolic changes in alkalosis

"AlK-loss, AlCa-loss":

There is loss of hypokalemia and hypocalcemia in state of alkalosis.

Allopurinol:

STORE

- S - Stones (history of renal stones)
- T - Tophaceous gout (chronic)
- O - Over-producers of urate
- R - renal disease
- E - Elderly

Bonus: Probenecid indications are basically the opposite of STORE (no renal stone history, etc.).

Dialysis indications

HAVE PEE:

- Hyperkalemia (refractory)
- Acidosis (refractory)
- Volume overload
- Elevated BUN (> 36 mM)
- Pericarditis
- Encephalopathy
- Edema (pulmonary)

Renal failure (acute): management

Manage AEIOU:

- Anemia/ Acidosis
- Electrolyte and fluids
- Infections
- Other measures (e.g., nutrition, nausea, vomiting)
- Uremia

SIADH: causes

SIADH:

- Surgery
- Intracranial: infection, head injury, CVA
- Alveolar: Ca, pus
- Drugs: opiates, antiepileptics, cytotoxic, anti-psychotics
- Hormonal: hypothyroid, low corticosteroid level

SIADH: diagnostic sign

Syndrome of INAPPropriate Anti-Diuretic Hormone:

- Increased
- Na (sodium)
- PP (urine)

SIADH is characterized by increased urinary sodium.

SIADH: major signs and symptoms

SIADH:

- Spasms
- Isn't any pitting edema (key DDx)
- Anorexia
- Disorientation (and other psychoses)
- Hyponatremia

Eosinophilia: differential

NAACP:

- Neoplasm
- Allergy/ Asthma
- Addison's disease
- Collagen vascular diseases
- Parasites

Polycythemia Rubra Vera (PRV): common symptoms

PRV:

- Plethora/ Pruritis
- Ringing in ears
- Visual blurriness

SLE: factors that make SLE active

UV PRISM:

- UV (sunshine)
- Pregnancy

- Reduced drug (e.g., steroid)
- Infection
- Stress
- More drug

Splenomegaly: causes

CHICAGO:

- Cancer
- Hemolytic Anemia
- Infection
- Congestion (portal hypertension)
- Autoimmune (RA, SLE)
- Glycogen storage disorders
- Other (amyloidosis)

Horner's syndrome: components

SAMPLE:

- Sympathetic chain injury
- Anhidrosis
- Miosis
- Ptosis
- Loss of ciliospinal reflex
- Enophthalmos

Lethargy, malaise causes

FATIGUED:

- Fat/ Food (poor diet)
- Anemia
- Tumor
- Infection (HIV, endocarditis)
- General joint or liver disease
- Uremia
- Endocrine (Addison's, myxedema) Diabetes/ Depression/ Drugs

Behcet's Syndrome:

PROSE:

- P- Pathergy test (i/d saline injection)
- R- Recurrent genital ulceration
- - Oral ulceration (recurrent)
- S - Skin lesions
- E - Eye lesions

ICU management:

A to Z

- A - Asepsis
- B - Bed sore/ Breathing/ Blood pressure C: Circulation/ encourage
- C- Coughing and Consciousness
- D - Drains
- E - ECG
- F - Fluid status
- G - GI losses/ Gag reflex
- H - Head positioning/ Height
- I - Insensible losses
- J - Jugular venous pulse
- K - Kindness
- L - Limb care/ Label
- M - Mouth care
- N - Nociception/ Nutrition
- - Oxygenation/ Orient the patient
- P - Pulse/ Peristalsis/ Physiotherapy Q: Quiet surroundings
- R - Respiratory rate/ Restraint S: Stress ulcer/ Suctioning
- T - Temperature
- U - Urine
- V - Ventilator
- W - Wounds/ Weight
- X - Xerosis
- Y -
- Z - Zestful care of the patient

Left iliac fossa: causes of pain

SUPER CLOT:

- Sigmoid diverticulitis
- Uteric colic
- PID
- Ectopic pregnancy

- Rectus sheath haematoma
- Colorectal carcinoma
- Left sided lower love pneumonia
- Ovarian cyst (rupture, torture)
- Threatened abortion/ Testicular torsion

Acute stridor: Differential

ABCDEFGH:

<u>With fever:</u>

- Abscess
- Bacterial tracheitis
- Croup
- Diphtheria
- Epiglottitis

<u>Without fever:</u>

- Foreign body
- Gas (Toxic Gas)
- Hypersensitivity

Bronchiectasis: causes

A SICK AIRWAY:

- Airway lesion, chronic obstruction
- Sequestration
- Infection, inflammation
- Cystic fibrosis
- Kartagener syndrome
- Allergic bronchopulmonary aspergillosis
- Immunodeficiencies (hypogammaglobinemia, myeloma, lymphoma)
- Reflux, inhalation injury
- William Campbell syndrome (and other congenital)
- Aspiration
- Yellow nail syndrome/ Young syndrome

Bronchiectasis: differential

BRONCHIECTASIS:

- Bronchial cyst
- Repeated gastric acid aspiration
- Or due to foreign bodies
- Necrotizing pneumonia
- Chemical corrosive substances
- Hypogammaglobulinemia
- Immotile cilia syndrome
- Eosinophilia (pulmonary)
- Cystic fibrosis
- Tuberculosis (primary)
- Atopic bronchial asthma
- Streptococcal pneumonia
- In Young's syndrome
- Staphylococcal pneumonia

Hemoptysis: Causes

HEMOPTYSIS:

- Hemorrhagic diathesis
- Edema [LVF due to mitral stenosis]
- Malignancy
- Others [e.g.: vasculitis]
- Pulmonary vascular abnormalities
- Trauma
- Your treatment [anticoagulants]
- SLE
- Infarction in lungs
- Septic

Pleural effusion: Investigations

PLEURA:

- Pleural fluid (thoracentesis)
- Lung, pleural biopsy
- ESR
- Ultrasound
- Radiogram
- Analysis of blood

Pulmonary edema: treatment

LMNOP:

- Lasix
- Morphine
- Nitrates (NTG)
- Oxygen
- Position (upright vs. flat)

Pulmonary edema: Treatments

MAD DOG:

- Morphine
- Aminophylline
- Digitalis
- Diuretics
- Oxygen
- Gases in blood (ABG's)

Pulmonary fibrosis: Causes

SCAR:

Upper lobe:

- Silicosis/ Sarcoidosis
- Coal worker pneumoconiosis
- Ankylosing spondylitis
- Radiation

Lower lobe:

- Systemic sclerosis
- Cryptogenic fibrosing alveolitis
- Asbestosis
- Rheumatoid arthritis

Wheezing: Causes

ASTHMA:

- Asthma

- Small airways disease
- Tracheal obstruction
- Heart failure
- Masto cytosis or carcinoid
- Anaphylaxis or allergy

Back Trouble causes

O, VERSALIUS (Vesalius was the name of a famous physician):

- Osteomyelitis
- Vertebral fracture
- Extraspinal tumor
- Spondylolisthesis
- Ankylosing spondylitis
- Lumbar disk increase
- Intraspinal tumor
- Unhappiness
- Stress

Chapter 4:   Neurology Mnemonics

Alzheimer's Disease – Symptoms

5 A's

- Anomia (can't remember names of things)
- Apraxia (using objects inappropriately)
- Aphasia (unable to express feelings with voice)
- Amnesia (memory loss)
- Agnosia (can't recognize familiar senses, such as taste, sounds, etc.)

Alzheimer's disease is a progressive and degenerative form of dementia. These patients often can't remember the names of things, can't recognize familiar senses and have a general loss of memory. They also have a difficult time using objects appropriately and have trouble expressing their feelings through their voice. These symptoms usually start out mild and may come and go. But they get worse as time goes by.

Bipolar Disorder – Depressive

DEAD SWAMP

- Depressed mood
- Energy loss
- Anhedonia
- Death thoughts (suicide)
- Sleep disturbances
- Worthlessness
- Appetite loss
- Mentation decreased
- Psychomotor - agitation

Bipolar disorder is characterized by changing periods of manic behavior and depressive behavior. In the depressive phase, these patients have suicidal thoughts, are easily agitated, and are unable to concentrate. They often lack interest in things, have feelings of guilt and a loss of appetite. They can be slow-moving and have a lack of energy.

Bipolar Disorder – Manic Episodes

FIDGETS

- Flight of ideas
- Indiscretion, Insomnia

- Distractibility
- Grandiosity
- Extra activity
- Talkative
- Sleep deficit

Bipolar disorder is characterized by changing periods of manic behavior and depressive behavior. In the manic phase, these patients can't seem to sit still. They are easily distracted, very talkative, and go from idea to idea. They often have delusions of grandiosity and have trouble getting to sleep.

Cranial Nerves – Innervation

Some Say Marry Money, But My Brother Says Big Books Matter Most

- Sensory
- Sensory
- Motor
- Motor
- Both
- Motor
- Both
- Sensory
- Both
- Both
- Motor
- Motor

CVA – Symptoms

BE FAST

- Balance (uncoordinated movements)
- Eyes (blurry vision)
- Facial Droop
- Arm weakness
- Speech slurred
- Tachycardia

Patients who are having a stroke don't usually know what's happening to them. This is why it is so important for us to recognize the symptoms quickly. Obvious signs are slurred speech, facial droop, and weakness on one side of the body. They may also have blurred vision and a high heart rate. Because of the weakness on one side, you may also see problems with their balance.

Dementia – Differential Diagnosis

DEMENTIA

- Drugs and Alcohol
- Eyes and Ears
- Metabolic and Endocrine disorders
- Emotional disorders
- Neurologic disorders
- Tumors and Trauma
- Infection
- Arteriovascular disease

Dementia represents many neurological disorders that are progressive and affect the ability to think and remember things. Some examples include Alzheimer's disease, vascular dementia, and Parkinson's dementia. Before you classify someone with such diseases, it's important to make a differential diagnosis to rule out other causes. Make sure it's not drugs, alcohol, infection, a tumor, the trauma of some sort, or arteriovascular disease. Check for problems with vision and hearing to make sure something like that isn't making them seem demented. Some metabolic, endocrine and other neurological disorders can also mimic dementia.

Glasgow Coma Scale (GCS)

A total score of 15 Possible (Eyes, Motor, Verbal)

Eye Opening – 4 Eyes (with glasses)

Motor – V6 Engine

Verbal – Jackson 5

EYES (4 Possible Points)

1. Eyes are shut (no response)
2. "Yikes" (eyes open to pain)
3. Ears (eyes open to voice)
4. Spontaneous eye-opening

Motor (OLDBEN – 6 Possible Points)

1. Obeys Commands
2. Localizes to pain
3. Draws away (withdraws from pain)
4. bend (flexion/decorticate response to pain)
5. Extension (decereberate response to pain)
6. No response

<u>Verbal (VOWEL - 5 Possible Points)</u>

1. Voiceless
2. Obscure (incomprehensible)
3. Weird words (Inappropriate words)
4. Erratic (confusing words)
5. Legit (normal)

Increased Intracranial Pressure (ICP) – Symptoms

Cushing's Triad (Hypertension, Bradycardia, Irregular Respirations) is easy to remember with this mnemonic:

RIB

- Respirations Irregular/Decreased
- Increased BP (Hypertension)
- Bradycardia

When there is an excessive cerebrospinal fluid in the brain and spinal cord, the intracranial pressure will increase. This can be due to various reasons but will often cause hypertension, bradycardia, and irregular respirations. Collectively, this is known as Cushing's Triad.

Increased Intracranial Pressure (ICP) – Treatment

MOCHA MOM

- Monitor ICP
- Osmotic diuretics
- Corticosteroids
- Hyperventilate
- Antipyretics
- Muscle relaxants
- Oxygen
- Maintain CO and cerebral perfusion

When there is an excessive cerebrospinal fluid in the brain and spinal cord, the intracranial pressure will increase. This can result in various reasons but can be treated with hyperventilation, osmotic diuretics, oxygen, muscle relaxants, antipyretics, and corticosteroids. While treating, make sure you are vigilant in monitoring intracranial pressure changes. Try to maintain the cardiac output and cerebral perfusion when using these modalities.

Meningitis – Signs/Symptoms

SHIT HAPPENS

- Seizures
- High temp (fever)
- Impaired (confused)
- Tired
- Headache
- Altered mental status
- Photophobia
- Petechiae on trunk/extremities
- Emesis
- Neck stiffness
- Sensitivity to sound

Meningitis is when the brain and spinal cord become inflamed. The culprit is usually infection, viral or bacterial. Some common symptoms include seizures, fever, confusion, tiredness, headache, photophobia (sensitivity to light), nausea, neck stiffness, sensitivity to sounds, and petechiae on the trunk and extremities. A bacterial infection is usually much worse and progresses very quickly. Antibiotics must be given in addition to supportive measures. For a viral infection, antivirals may be given but aren't typically successful. This form of meningitis will just have to run its course while the symptoms are treated.

Maslow's Hierarchy of Needs

People Should Live Every Second (Basic to a higher level)

- Self-Actualization
- Esteem
- Love/belonging
- Safety
- Physiological

For Maslow's Hierarchy of Needs, start from the bottom (the most basic) and work your way up. In general, most of us go through life in this order, not moving on to the next level until the previous one has been realized. Physiological needs are considered the most basic, such as food, water, and shelter. Once these have been met, a person can then be compelled to seek out safety, including physical, emotional, health, and financial. Once safety is at a level a person is comfortable with, they will begin to seek out love and the feeling of belonging to a group (family, friends, co-workers). The next level is esteem, in which people aim to achieve things that bring self-esteem and esteem from others. Finally, self-actualization is at the top of the hierarchy. Usually, this can't be attained until the levels below are realized. Here, people are trying to attain something that will bring ultimate satisfaction and a feeling of accomplishment. For example, a goal is achieved, a soulmate is found, happiness is obtained. This level could be anything and is really up to each individual person to decide what they are going for.

Multiple Sclerosis – Symptoms

DANISH

- Dysdiadochokinesia
- Ataxia
- Nystagmus
- Intentional tremor
- Scanning speech
- Hypotonia

Multiple Sclerosis is a disease that happens when the covers that insulate the nerve cells in the spinal cord and the brain become damaged. Because of this, it is considered a demyelinating disease. Symptoms can vary from patient to patient and depend on the progression of the disease. Some of the things you might see include urinary retention, weakness, constipation, blurred vision, and tinnitus (ringing ears). Many patients experience dysdiadochokinesia, which means they aren't able to make rapid, alternating movements. Ataxia means they don't have the coordination of muscle movements. Nystagmus is involuntary eye movement. Intentional tremor is a low-frequency tremor in which the person attempts to move an extremity to a certain spot but goes slightly farther or shorter. Scanning speech refers to words that get broken up into syllables with a clear pause in many cases. Hypotonia is decreased muscle tone.

Neurogenic Shock – Causes

BAMS

- Brain injury
- Anesthesia (spinal)
- Meds
- Spinal cord injury (above T5)

In neurogenic shock, the autonomic pathways of the spinal cord are interrupted, leading to hypotension and often bradycardia. Some of the causes include brain injury, certain medications, spinal cord injuries that occur above T5, and spinal anesthesia (too much). Decreased systemic vascular resistance and loss of sympathetic tone are the result. If the problem isn't spotted and corrected quickly, then it can lead to organ damage and eventually death.

Neurogenic Shock – Symptoms

BUSHED

- Bradycardia
- Unopposed vagal activity
- Skin warm and flushed
- Hypotension

- Erection (priapism – prolonged erection without arousal)
- Decreased SVR

In neurogenic shock, the autonomic pathways of the spinal cord are interrupted, leading to hypotension and often bradycardia. This is caused by the decreased systemic vascular resistance and loss of sympathetic tone. If the problem isn't spotted and corrected quickly, then it can lead to organ damage and eventually death. In addition, other common symptoms include flushed skin, prolonged erection without arousal, and unopposed vagal activity (due to the loss of sympathetic tone).

Parkinson's Disease – Symptoms

SMART

- Shuffling gait
- Mask-like facies
- Akinesia, bradykinesia
- Rigidity
- Tremor

Parkinson's disease is caused by a lack of dopamine that is normally produced by neurons in the brain. When these neurons become damaged, as is the case in Parkinson's, they are unable to produce dopamine. This progressive disease causes a range of symptoms but can eventually lead to tremor, rigidity, shuffling gait, akinesia/bradykinesia, and mask-like facies. Bradykinesia is a very slow voluntary movement, while akinesia is the lack of control of voluntary movements. Mask-like facies refers to the lack of facial expression these patients often exhibit. Because they show no emotion, it often looks like a mask instead of a face.

Pupils – Exam

PERRLA

- Pupils
- Equal
- Round and
- Reactive to
- Light and
- Accommodation

When performing an eye exam, use PERRLA to make sure you don't forget to check something. In regard to the pupils, you want to make sure they are equal in size, round (not misshapen), and reactive to light (constrict), and accommodation. Accommodation means the pupils should constrict when focusing on a near object and dilate when focusing on an object that is farther away. They should constrict in response to light and dilate in response to darkness.

Pupils – Mydriasis (Dilation) Causes

AAA South

- Antihistamines
- Antidepressants
- Anticholinergics (e.g., Atropine)
- Sympathomimetics

Aside from naturally reacting to light and darkness, some medications can cause the pupils to dilate and constrict. Medications that can cause pupil dilation (mydriasis) include antihistamines (diphenhydramine), antidepressants (amitriptyline), anticholinergics (Atropine), and sympathomimetics (pseudoephedrine). Other culprits include some anti-seizure medications, Botox, Parkinson's medications, and anti-nausea medications.

Pupils – Miosis (Constriction) Causes

COMPLAINS

- Clonidine
- Opiates
- Mushrooms/Muscarinic agents
- Phenothiazines
- Lomotil
- Asleep
- Insecticides
- Narcotics
- Stroke, Sedatives

Aside from naturally reacting to light and darkness, some outside influences can cause the pupils to dilate and constrict. Some things that can cause pupil constriction (miosis) include clonidine, opiates, mushrooms, phenothiazines (Compazine), Lomotil, insecticides, narcotics, stroke, sedatives, and the simple act of being asleep.

Schizophrenia – Symptoms

The CRAP rolls DOWNHILL

- Changes in personality
- Religiosity
- Autism
- Peculiar behavior
- Delusions
- Often disorganized

- Withdrawn
- Negativism
- Hallucinations/Hypersensitivity to sound, sight, and smell
- Indifferent
- Loss of ego
- Lack of social awareness

Schizophrenia is a disease in which people see reality differently. This condition is characterized by changes in personality, peculiar behavior, delusions, hallucinations, and lack of social awareness. They often have strong feelings toward religion, and they can be disorganized. They are usually withdrawn, have a negative outlook, loss of ego, and are hypersensitive to certain senses. There is sometimes a correlation between some forms of autism and schizophrenia.

Chapter 5: Anesthesia Mnemonics

Gas Cylinders – Amount Remaining

The amount remaining in the cylinder can be determined by the reading on the pressure gauge with these 4 gases:

NOAH

- Nitrogen
- Oxygen
- Air
- Helium

If gases are in liquid form in the cylinder, then the amount remaining cannot be ascertained simply by reading the pressure gauge. However, nitrogen, oxygen, air, and helium are all gases that are not in liquid form in high-pressure cylinders. Therefore, you can determine the amount remaining by reading the pressure gauge.

Orbital Muscles

IS SLIM

- Inferior Rectus
- Superior Rectus

- Superior Oblique
- Lateral Rectus
- Inferior Oblique
- Medial Rectus

Inferior Rectus: look down (Cranial nerve III – oculomotor)

Superior Rectus: lookup (Cranial nerve III – oculomotor)

Superior Oblique: look in and down (Cranial nerve IV – trochlear)

Lateral Rectus: look outward (Cranial nerve VI – abducens)

Inferior Oblique: look out and up (Cranial nerve III – oculomotor)

Medial Rectus: look inward (Cranial nerve III – oculomotor)

Aldrete's Scoring System – Criteria

ARCCC

- Activity
- Respiration
- Circulation
- Consciousness
- Color

Aldrete's scoring system is used by the post-anesthesia care unit to determine when it's safe to discharge the patient to the next phase. The five criteria that comprise this system include activity, respiration, circulation, consciousness, and color. Each of these is worth 0 to 2 points, and patients can be discharged when their score is greater than 8. However, they may be kept longer if the nurses and doctors deem it necessary.

Medical Negligence Action - Elements

Dumb Boys Don't Call.

- Duty
- Breach of Duty
- Damage
- Cause

If a plaintiff brings forth a medical negligence action, they must prove that duty, breach of duty, damage, and 'cause' all existed in their case. Duty means that a reasonable standard of care was expected. Breach of duty means that this standard was not met in some way. Damage means that physical or emotional injury occurred. Cause means that the damage was caused by the defendant. The damage to the plaintiff must be a direct result of the defendant's action.

MRI Contraindications – Implanted Devices

CAB

- Cardiac pacemakers
- AICD
- Biological pumps

Any object with a high susceptibility to magnetization could place the patient or that object at risk during an MRI. Biological pumps, such as implanted pain pumps and insulin pumps, may get damaged or cause harm to the patient. The same can be said for pacemakers and AICDs, which may convert to asynchronous mode, be deactivated, or get switch damage. MRIs may also be contraindicated in patients with vascular clips, stents, and wire-spiraled endotracheal tubes.

Soda Lime Exhaustion - Indicators

FAITH

- Flushed dry skin
- Absorbent turns color
- Inspired CO2 concentration increases
- Tachycardia
- Hypertension

When the patient is showing any signs of increased CO2 production, then you might want to take a look at your soda lime canister to see if it needs to be changed. Common signs of soda-lime exhaustion include flushed dry skin, tachycardia, and hypertension. The easiest way to tell, though, is by looking at your CO2 waveform and the canister itself. If the patient is rebreathing CO2, the absorbent has changed color, and there is a large amount of condensation in the canister, then the soda-lime has probably been exhausted. Get a new one!

Awareness During Anesthesia – Increased Risk

PITA (Pain In The Ass)

- Provider abuse of anesthetic drugs
- Inhalational agent not turned on/empty vaporizer
- TIVA not begun or failure of the device
- Anesthesia discontinued too early

Awareness during anesthesia can be a very scary thing for our patients. One of the most asked questions in the pre-operative area is, "how do you know if I'm asleep enough?" Although a rare occurrence, there are some things that may increase the risk of awareness. If the anesthesia provider is abusing the anesthetics, then they may charge some drugs to the patient but never administer them instead of pocketing them for later. The anesthetist may forget to turn on the gas or simply forget to fill the vaporizer. Another problem may occur during a TIVA when gas can't be used. After induction, the IV meds may be forgotten (since the anesthetist is used to turning on the gas rather than starting a pump). Lastly, anesthesia may be discontinued too early. As the surgery is ending, the anesthetist may cut the gas too early in trying to achieve "the perfect wakeup."

Volatile Anesthetics – Renal Changes

RUG

- Renal blood flow
- Urine output
- Glomerular filtration rate

Volatile anesthetics can affect many body systems in various ways, and the kidneys are no exception. They can cause decreases in renal blood flow, urine output, and glomerular filtration rate. Desflurane may be a better choice in patients with already impaired renal function.

Gamma Amino Butyric Acid Type A (GABAA) Receptor – Ligand Binding Sites

GABAS Possessive Binding Places

- G
- Anesthetics
- Barbiturates
- Alcohol
- Steroids

- Propofol
- Benzodiazepines
- Picrotoxin

We should all be familiar with the name gamma-aminobutyric acid (GABA) since it is believed to have much to do with the function of anesthesia. If you look closely, you'll see that five of these sites involve anesthesia. GABA Type A ligand binding sites include anesthetics, barbiturates, alcohol, steroids, Propofol, benzodiazepines, and picrotoxin.

Heat Loss – Causes (Most to Least)

Really Cover Every Corner

- Radiation
- Convection
- Evaporation
- Conduction

As anesthesia providers, we're responsible for the maintenance of patient temperature, making sure they don't get hypothermic. Therefore, it's important to know how heat is lost so we can figure out ways to stop it. During anesthesia, heat is mostly lost through radiation, which is the transfer of heat from the body to other cooler things nearby. The patient loses heat when the ambient temperature in the operating room is too low. Convection happens when forced-air flows over exposed skin and removes heat along with it. Heat is lost by evaporation through the use of surgical prep solutions and open cavities in the body. Conduction is when the heat gets transferred from the body to a surface it is in contact with, such as the cold operating room bed.

Volatile Inhaled Agents – Trade Names

HF – Hepatic Failure; EE – Evil Empire; IF – I Farted; DS – Dark Side; SU – Suck Up

- Halothane is Fluothane™
- Enflurane is Ethrane™
- Isoflurane is Forane™
- Desflurane is Suprane™
- Sevoflurane is Ultane™

Nitrous Oxide (N2O) – Side Effects

CACA

- Congenital anomalies
- Aplastic anemia
- CNS toxicity
- Abortion (Spontaneous)

As we all know, nitrous oxide isn't without serious side effects. For instance, it is known to cause nausea and can also get trapped in closed air spaces, so it should be avoided in certain patients. It may cause spontaneous abortion or congenital anomalies, so avoid or use caution in pregnant patients, particularly during organogenesis. Nitrous oxides could also cause central nervous system toxicity and aplastic anemia. Although it can be a very useful drug, be cautious when administering it and make sure you think before you turn that dial.

Anesthetic Brain Uptake – Dependent Factors

Anesthesia Is Briskly Changing

- Alveolar Ventilation
- Inspired Concentration
- Blood Solubility
- Cardiac Output

The uptake of volatile anesthetics by the brain is dependent upon several factors. The higher the alveolar ventilation, the faster the uptake. The more you increase the inspired concentration, the faster the uptake. The more blood soluble a gas is, the slower the uptake due to the slower rise in alveolar partial pressure. Finally, when a patient has a lower cardiac output, it increases the uptake to the brain.

HIGHER Alveolar ventilation = FASTER uptake

HIGHER Inspired concentration = FASTER uptake

HIGHER Blood solubility = SLOWER uptake

HIGHER Cardiac output = SLOWER uptake

Chapter 6: Head & Neck

Cranium

Scalp: layers

SCALP

- S skin
- C connective tissue
- A aponeurosis
- L loose connective tissue
- P periosteum

Scalp: nerve supply

GLASS:

- Greater occipital/ Greater auricular
- Lesser occipital
- Auriculotemporal
- Supratrochlear
- Supraorbital

Occipitofrontalis

Frontalis

- O: aponeurosis
- I: the skin of the eyebrows
- A: it elevates the eyebrows and wrinkles the forehead
- N: temporal branches of the facial nerve (VII)
- Occipitalis
- O: superior nuchal line
- I: aponeurosis
- A: elevates the eyebrows and wrinkles the forehead
- N: posterior auricular branch of the facial nerve (VII)
- NB: the frontalis and occipitalis muscles are two bellies of the occipitofrontalis muscle, also known as epicranius m.

Cavernous sinus: relations

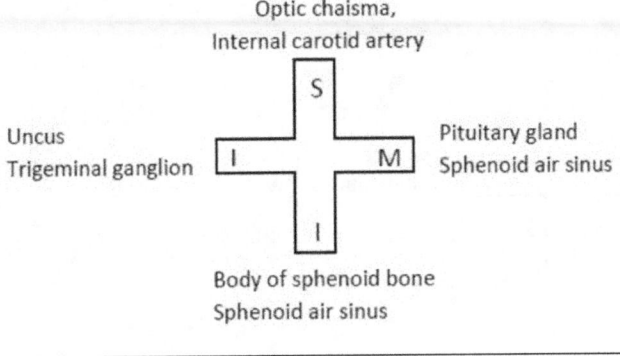

Cavernous sinus: communications

Below stated the anterior, posterior, inferior & superior communications. Medially, the 2 cavernous sinuses communicate with each other by 3 intercavernous sinuses.

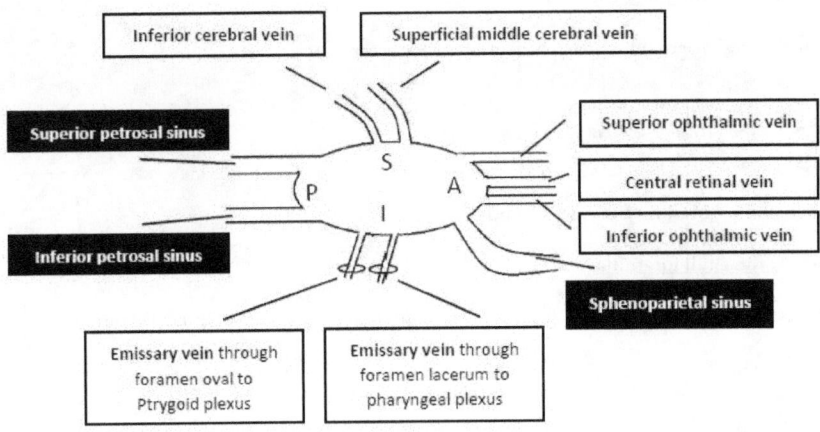

Pituitary gland: relations

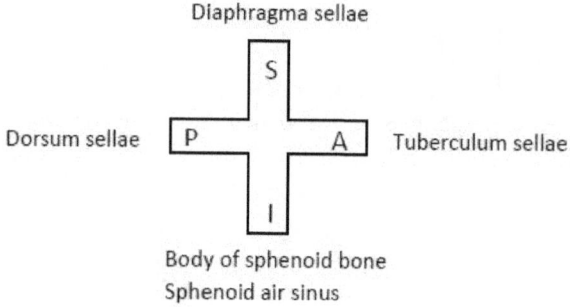

Orbit: bones of medial wall

"My Little Eye Sits in orbit":

- Maxilla (frontal process)
- Lacrimal
- Ethmoid
- Sphenoid (body)

Ear: bones of the inner ear

Describes the shape and relative position of the inner ear bones:

- *Take a Hammer*: Malleus
- *Hit an Indian Elephant*: Incus
- *It puts its foot in a stirrup*: Stapes

Alternatively: **"Mailing Includes Stamps."**

Base of the skull foramina

ROS is a well-known mnemonic for the 3 important foramina of the middle cranial fossa.

- Rotunda
- Ovale
- Spinosum

Foramen	From	Passing[1]	To
Cribriform plate	Anterior cranial fossa	Olfactory (CN1[2])	Ethmoid air cells – nasal cavity
Optic		Optic (CN2) Ophthalmic artery	Orbit
Superior orbital fissure	Middle cranial fossa	Oculomotor (CN3) Trochlear (CN4) Ophthalmic div. of trigeminal (CN5a) Abducent (CN6)	Orbit (posteromedial)
Rotundum		Maxillary div. of trigeminal (CN5b)	Inferior orbital fissure – pterygopalatine fossa
Ovale		Maxillary div. of trigeminal (CN5b)	The other side of the sphenoid bone medial to tempromandibular joint
Spinosum		Middle meningeal artery Meningeal branch of mandibular nerve	
Lacerum		Part of the course of internal carotid artery	Between body of sphenoid and basal part of occipital bone
Internal auditory meatus	Posterior cranial fossa	Fascial (CN7) Vestibulocochlear (CN8) Labyrinthine artery	Through petrous part of temporal bone, via middle ear to external auditory meatus
Hypoglossal		Hypoglossal (CN12)	Near articular facet of atlanto-occipital
Jugular		Glossopharyngeal (CN9) Vagus (CN10) Accessory (CN11) Sigmoid sinus to Internal jugular vein	Medial to styloid process
Magnum		Medulla oblongata Spinal root of accessory n. Vertebral artery Anterior & posterior spinal arteries	Central vertebral canal

Foramina: connections & structures passing

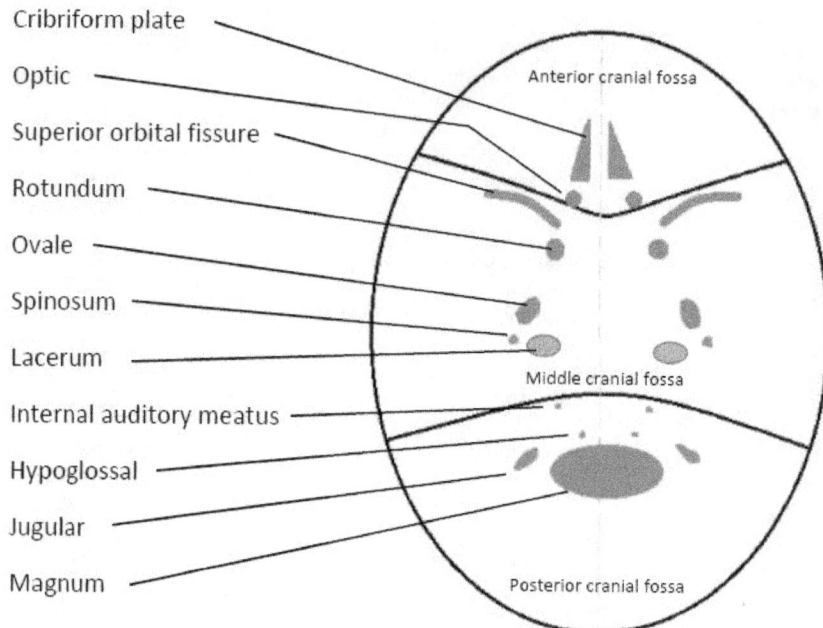

1 Only major structure are mentioned here
2 CN = cranial nerve

Foramen ovale contents

OVALE:

- Otic ganglion (just inferior)
- V3 cranial nerve
- Accessory meningeal artery
- Lesser petrosal nerve
- Emissary's veins

Another mnemonic

MALE

- Mandibular nerve
- Accessory meningeal artery
- Lesser petrosal nerve
- Emissary's veins

Foramen magnum

VAMPIRE

- Vertebral artery
- Anterior spinal artery
- Medulla oblongata
- Posterior Spinal artery
- It's covering (meninges covering of the medulla)
- Root of accessory nerve (spinal root)
- Enough

Foramen magnum

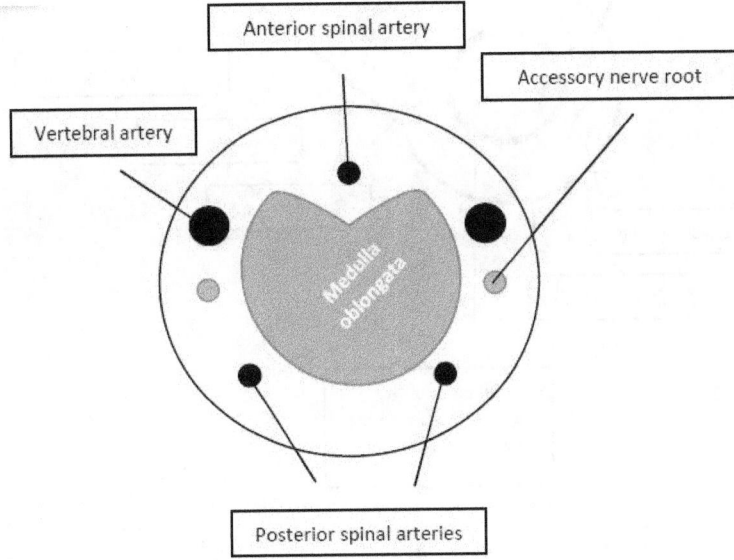

Foramina of Luschka and Magendie

The roof of the 4th ventricle has three foramina: the medial foramen of Magendie and two foramens of Luschka. They transmit the cerebrospinal fluid into the subarachnoid space.

The locations of these foramina are:

- Magendie Medial
- Luschka Lateral

Jugular foramen

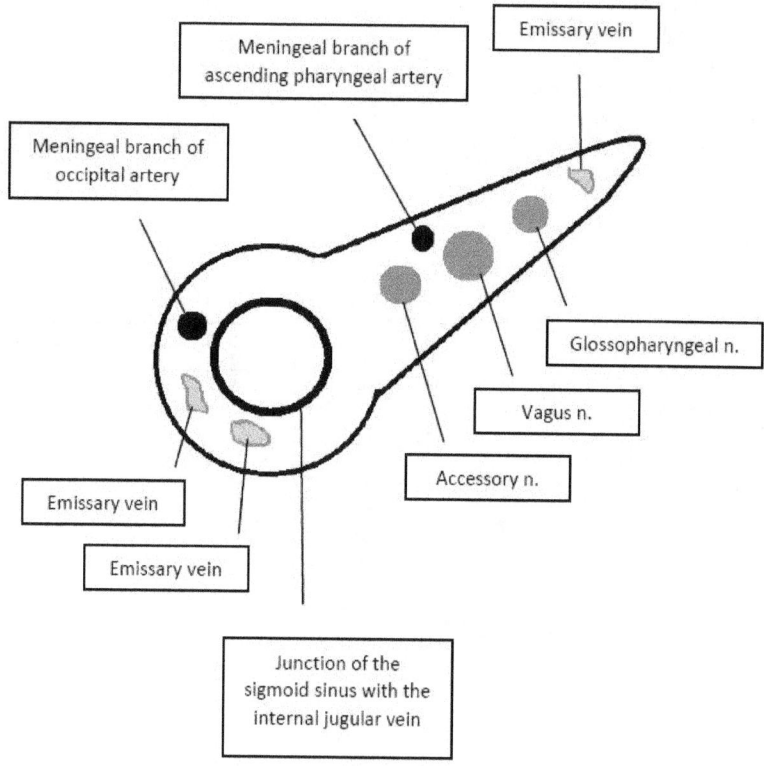

Superior orbital fissure: structures passing through

"Live Free To See Absolutely No Insult":

- Lacrimal nerve
- Frontal nerve
- Trochlear nerve
- Superior branch of Oculomotor nerve
- Abducent nerve
- Nasociliary nerve
- Inferior branch of Oculomotor nerve

Inferior orbital fissures: Structures passing through

"ZIME"

- Zygomatic nerve
- Infraorbital vessels
- Maxillary nerve
- Emissary's vein

Cranial nerves and eye movements

SALT ME DOWN:

S- Six

A- Abducts

L- Laterally

T- Trochlear acts

Medially Down.

Oculomotor nerve is responsible for everything else.

CN6 = Abducent > supply the lateral rectus only, so abducts the eye.

CN4 = Trochlear > supply the superior oblique only, so it depresses the eye (only when the eye is adducted or moving medially by the medial rectus.

CN3 = oculomotor > supply the other 4 muscles, so responsible for the rest of eye movements.

Orbit fissures & extraocular muscles

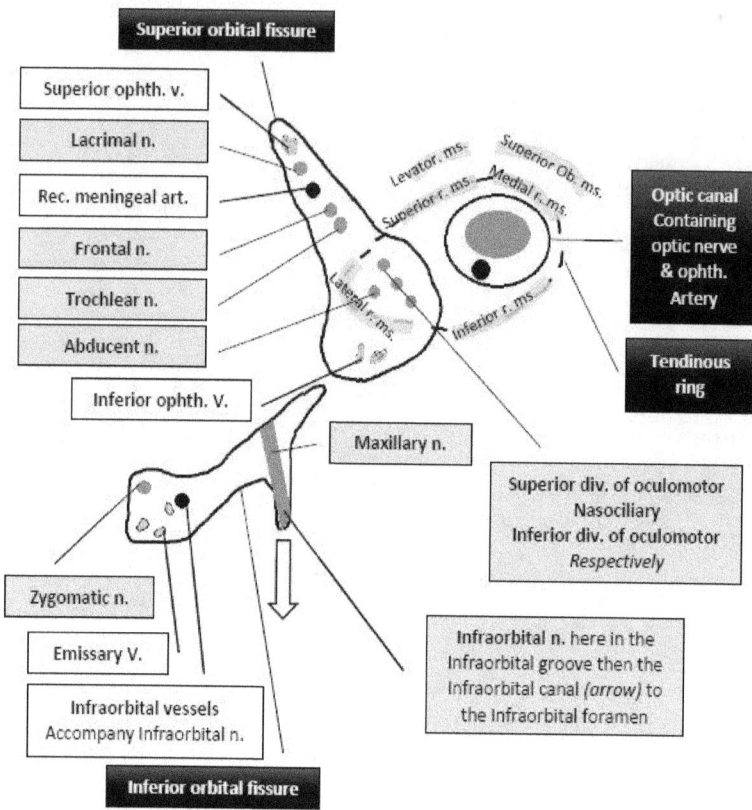

Important foramina content

"Max Returns Mandy's Ovum… May Marry Spinster"

- MAX = Maxillary nerve
- Returns foramen = Rotundum
- Mandy's = Mandibular nerve
- Ovum = foramen Ovale
- May Marry = Middle Meningeal Artery
- Spinster = foramen Spinosum

Lacrimal nerve course

"Lacrimal's story of 8 L's":

The **lacrimal** nerve runs on the **Lateral** wall of orbit above the **Lateral** rectus. Then **Lets** communicating branch join in. Then supplies **Lacrimal gland**. Then **Leaves** it and supplies the **Lateral** upper eye **Lid**!

Brain lobes & its functions

The frontal contains prefrontal (emotions, personality) and precentral (primary and secondary motor) areas.

The parietal contains the primary and secondary somatosensory areas.

Temporal is primarily concerned with hearing and memory/learning.

The occipital contains the primary and secondary visual cortex.

The Limbic is the part of the brain responsible for behavior and emotions.

Cranial nerves: names & types

Names: Oh, Oh, Oh, To Take A Family Vacation! Go Vegas After Hours.

Sensory or motor: Some say marry money, but my brother says big brain matter more.

Nr.	Cranial Nerves	Mnemonic	Type
I	Olfactory	Oh	Some (Sensory)
II	Optic	Oh	Say (Sensory)
III	Oculomotor	Oh	Marry (primarily Motor)
IV	Trochlear	To	Money, (primarily Motor)
V	Trigeminal	Try	But (Both)
VI	Abducent	A	My (primarily Motor)
VII	Facial	Family	Brother (Both)
VIII	Vestibulocochlear	Vacation	Says (Sensory)
IX	Glossopharyngeal	Go	Big (Both)
X	Vagus	Vegas	Brain (Both)
XI	Accessory Nerve	After	Matter (primarily Motor)
XII	Hypoglossal	Hours	More (primarily Motor)

Circle of Willis

Meet the weird Mr. Willis!

He has Eyes, hair, face, arms, legs, chest, and a penis

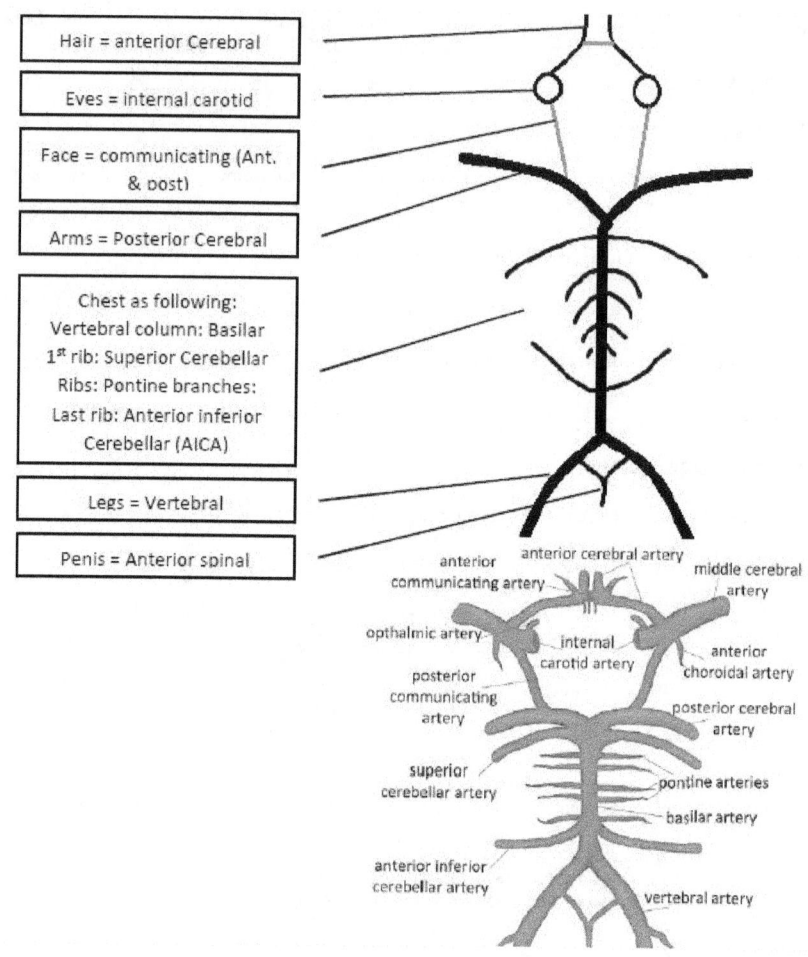

Hair = anterior Cerebral

Eyes = internal carotid

Face = communicating (Ant. & post)

Arms = Posterior Cerebral

Chest as following:
Vertebral column: Basilar
1st rib: Superior Cerebellar
Ribs: Pontine branches:
Last rib: Anterior inferior Cerebellar (AICA)

Legs = Vertebral

Penis = Anterior spinal

Don't you dare mock Mr. Willis unless you found your own Royal College of Surgeons, discover a circle of arteries in the base of the brain, and number the cranial nerves as we still do nowadays. Thomas Willis (1621 –1675)

Face & jaw

Facial nerve: branches after Stylomastoid foramen

"Tow Zombies Borrowed My Car":

Alternatively: "To Zanzibar By Motor Car"

From superior to inferior:

- Temporal branch
- Zygomatic branch
- Buccal branch
- Mandibular branch
- Cervical branch

Bell's palsy: symptoms

BELL's palsy:

- Blink reflex abnormal
- Earache
- Lacrimation [deficient, excess]
- Loss of taste
- Sudden onset
- Palsy of VII nerve muscles

Parotid gland – structures exiting its borders

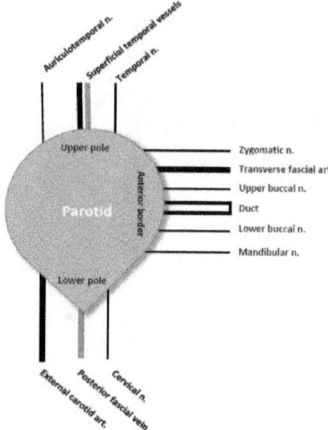

Muscles of mastication

Note: for all the four muscles, a branch is named after each muscle from the mandibular division of the trigeminal nerve (V).

Masseter

- O: zygomatic arch and zygomatic bone
- I: lateral surface of the ramus and angle of the mandible
- A: elevates the mandible

NB: a powerful chewing muscle

Temporalis

- O: temporal fossa and the temporal fascia
- I: the coronoid process of the mandible and the anterior surface of the ramus of the mandible
- A: elevates the mandible; retracts the mandible (posterior fibers)

NB: a powerful chewing muscle; a derivative of the first pharyngeal arch

Lateral pterygoid

- O: superior head: greater wing of the sphenoid bone; inferior head: lateral surface of the lateral pterygoid plate

- I: superior head: capsule and & articular disk of the temporomandibular joint; inferior head: neck of the mandible
- A: protracts the mandible; opens the mouth; active in grinding actions of chewing

NB: the only one of the muscles of mastication that opens the mouth; the superior head of lateral pterygoid is sometimes called sphenomeniscus due to its insertion into the disc of the temporomandibular joint

Medial pterygoid

- O: medial surface of the lateral pterygoid plate, the pyramidal process of the palatine bone, tuberosity of the maxilla
- I: medial surface of the ramus and angle of the mandible
- A: elevates and protracts the mandible

NB: this muscle mirrors the masseter m. in position and action with the ramus of the mandible between the two mm.

Facial bones

"Virgil Can Not Make My Pet Zebra Laugh!"

- Vomer
- Conchae
- Nasal
- Maxilla
- Mandible
- Palatine
- Zygomatic
- Lacrimal

Mandibular nerve innervated muscles

(Branchial arch 1 derivatives)

"M.D. My TV":

- Mastication [masseter, temporalis, pterygoids]
- Digastric [anterior belly]
- Mylohyoid tensor
- Tympani tensor
- Veli palatini

Extrinsic muscles of the tongue

(For pro soccer fans)

"Paris St. Germain's Hour":

- Palatoglossus
- Styloglossus
- Genioglossus
- Hyoglossus

NB. PSG is a French soccer team (foreign). Hence extrinsic comes to mind.

Three important muscles of the face

Buccinator

- O: pterygomandibular raphe, mandible, and the maxilla lateral to the molar teeth
- I: angle of the mouth and the lateral portion of the upper and lower lips
- A: pulls the corner of mouth laterally; presses the cheek against the teeth
- N: facial nerve (VII)

NB: although the buccinator is important in mastication, it is innervated by the buccal branch of the facial nerve and NOT by the buccal nerve from V3 (a sensory nerve)

Orbicularis Oris

- O: skin and fascia of lips and the area surrounding the lips
- I: skin and fascia of the lips
- A: purses the lips
- N: facial nerve (VII)

NB: the "kissing" muscle

Orbicularis oculi

- O: orbital part: medial orbital margin and the medial palpebral ligament; palpebral part: medial palpebral ligament
- I: orbital part: skin of the lateral cheek; palpebral part: lateral palpebral raphe
- A: closes the eyelids
- N: facial nerve (VII)

NB: activated involuntarily in the blink reflex; the palpebral part is active in normal blinking, and the orbital part is used to forcefully close the eye

Neck

Subclavian artery branches

"Very Tired Individuals Sip Strong Coffee Served Daily":

- Vertebral artery
- Thyrocervical trunk
- ---Inferior thyroid
- ---Superficial cervical
- ---Suprascapular
- Costocervical
- ---Superior intercostal
- ---Deep cervical

External carotid artery branches

"Some American Ladies Find Our Pyramids Most SaTisfactory":

Down and upwards

- Superior thyroid
- Ascending pharyngeal
- Lingual
- Facial
- Occipital
- Posterior auricular
- Maxillary
- Superficial Temporal

Carotid sheath contents

"I See 10 CC's in the IV"

- I See (I.C.) = Internal Carotid artery
- 10 = CN 10 (Vagus nerve)
- CC = Common Carotid artery
- IV = Internal Jugular Vein

Superior thyroid artery branches

"May I Softly Squeeze Charlie's Guitar?"

- Muscular

- Infrahyoid
- Superior laryngeal
- Sternomastoid
- Cricothyroid
- Glandular

External jugular vein: tributaries

PAST:

- Posterior external jugular vein
- Anterior jugular vein
- Suprascapular vein
- Transverse cervical vein

Six triangles of the neck – borders & content

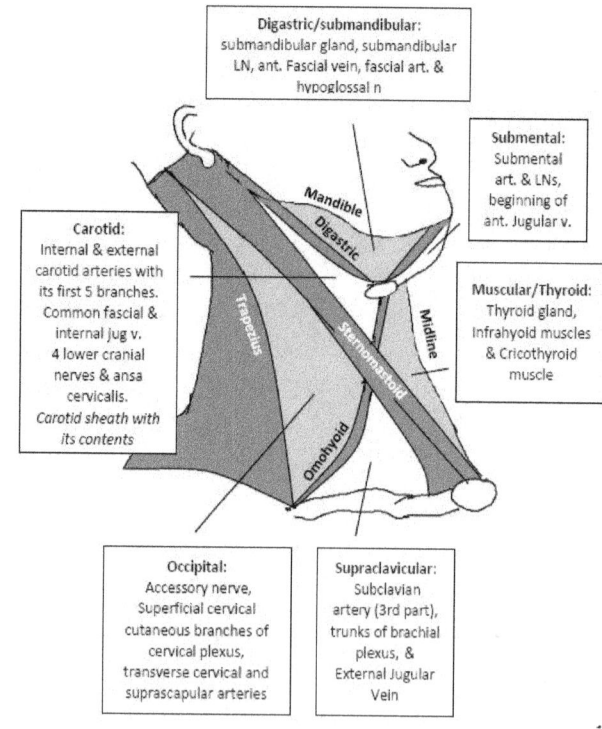

Cervical plexus: arrangement of the important cutaneous nerves

At the posterior border of the Sternomastoid.

"GLAST":

4 compass points: clockwise from the north on the right side of neck:

- Great auricular
- Lesser occipital
- Accessory nerve pops out between L and S
- Supraclavicular
- Transverse cervical

Ansa cervicalis nerves

"GHost THought Someone STupid SHot Irene":

- Geniohyoid
- Thyrohyoid
- Superior Omohyoid
- Sternothyroid
- Sternohyoid
- Inferior omohyoid

Horner's syndrome components

SPAM:

- Sunken eyeballs/ Sympathetic plexus (cervical) affected
- Ptosis
- Anhydrosis
- Miosis

Cervical plexus & ansa cervicalis

It is formed of ventral primary rami of spinal nerves C1-C4.

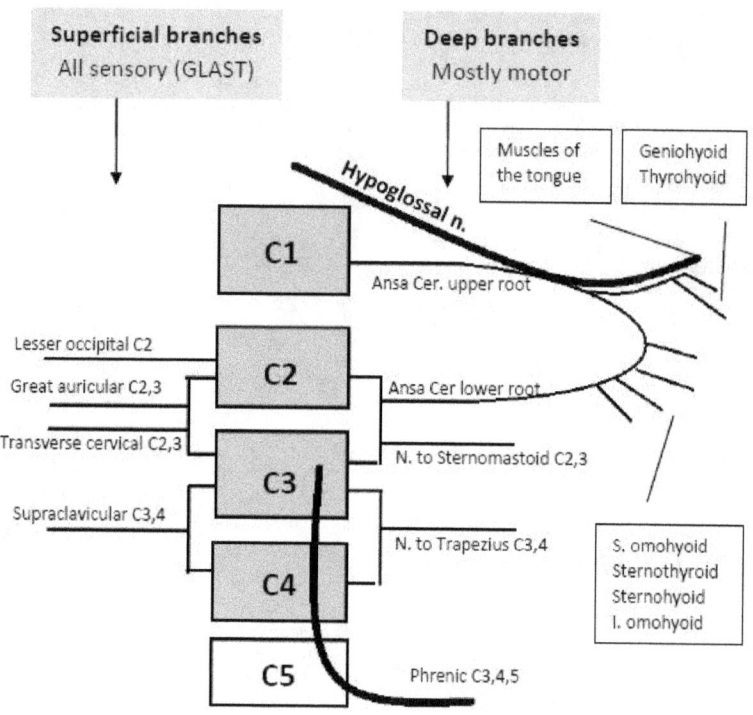

NB. Close association of the supraclavicular n. to the phrenic n. results in pain from the respiratory diaphragm referred to the shoulder C2,3 – e.g. in cholecystitis and acute myocardial ischemia pain are referred to rt. & lt. shoulders respectively.

Thyroid: isthmus location

It is the constricted midline connection between the lateral lobes of the thyroid gland.

"Rings 2, 3, 4 - make the isthmus floor":

- Isthmus overlies tracheal rings 2, 3, 4

Symptoms of hypothyroidism

Hypothyroidism is ten times more common in females & occurs mainly in middle life.

Mnemonic: MOM'S SO TIRED

- Memory loss
- Obesity
- Malar flush/Menorrhagia
- Slowness
- Skin and hair become dry
- Onset is gradual
- Tired
- Intolerance to cold
- Raised blood pressure
- Energy levels are low
- Depressed

Symptoms of hyperthyroidism

Mnemonic: SWEATING

- Sweating
- Weight loss
- Emotional liability
- Appetite is increased
- Tremor/Tachycardia due to AF
- Intolerance to heat/Irregular menstruation/Irritability
- Nervousness
- Goiter and Gastrointestinal problems (loose stools/diarrhea)

Conclusion

There's so much more to building a great memory than simply learning a few techniques. It's about making a lifestyle change. Nobody wants to have a superb memory for a few months and then go back to forgetting everything. Once you've started seeing results with your mnemonic techniques, it's in your best interest to set up a support system so that your memory journey ahead can be smooth, easy, and strong.

There are some things you can do to prepare for training your memory. They are:

- Meditation
- Getting into great sleep habits
- Physical exercise
- Family involvement

Those aren't all we can do to give our brain the best chance of learning, though. If you're implementing mnemonics strategies into your life on a daily basis, you're already developing new, healthy habits that will serve your memory well as you go.

Don't Stop Your Development

You're off to the best start you can be if you've implemented mnemonic techniques and are starting to reap the rewards. But if you stop here, you'll never achieve your full potential. Continuous improvement is essential. If you never move on from where you are right now, you're missing out on an amazing memory!

Here are some more ideas to start building a memory-centric lifestyle.

Build Your Memory Muscles

Just like building your physical muscles requires exercise and time, so too does your memory. You need to keep those memory muscles tough, and here are small but significant ways you can do that.

Train Daily

Inconsistency is the worst enemy of progress. Training daily is the minimum requirement in order to see startling progress. You can practice these tricks anywhere, anytime, no matter who's around you or what you're doing. There's no excuse!

Try one of these quick but effective exercises if you aren't sure exactly what to do:

- Memorize 4 details of people you encounter while out and about (observe now, recall later).
- Try to draw a mental map of where you are and how you get there.

You'll also notice there are other recommendations to gear your lifestyle towards being memory-friendly. Memory is like a puppy, in some ways—it thrives in a happy, healthy environment where it's taken care of, given room to play, and allowed plenty of exercise.

Socialize

This is referenced in many studies regarding Alzheimer's and how to prevent it (Diament, 2008). Despite being geared towards older persons, it's true for younger people too.

Socializing is something humans are designed to do (Shultz et al., 2011). It provides certain clear benefits, like:

- Increasing empathy (closely linked to memory)
- Exposure to various opinions—increase in intellect
- Opportunity for learning
- Create a support system

Just to clarify—I mean real, face-to-face socialization here. Social media has its place, but there's no substitute for the real thing.

Learn a New Skill or Hobby

Learning new skills stimulates your episodic and procedural memory, strengthening them in the process. Some skills are better than others at improving memory. Here are some recommended choices:

- **A Musical Instrument**

Music is a multi-faceted hobby. Not only will you be learning how to move your hands (and perhaps feet) in new ways, you'll possibly have to learn to move them independent of each other. You'll also need to learn how to read music or chords, how to keep timing, how to play with others, and possibly how to recognize notes by ear.

Music is one of those activities that involves more than one sense at a time, which may explain why it's so good for improving memory (Talamini et al., 2017).

- **A Foreign Language**

It's also the perfect chance to start implementing your new techniques. Don't be afraid to try it and use techniques to remember words. Association is a great one if you're learning a language that's not too different.

For example, "cat" in Italian is "gatto." You could equate this to a gate, and imagine a ginger sitting on your gate. Then, when you hear the word (in English or Italian) you automatically picture a cat on a gate, and so your mind finds "gatto."

Take a new course

Is there an online course you've had your heart set on? Whether it's business, hobby, or something random, learning something new stimulates the brain and gets neural pathways firing.

The course you pick can be anything. The memorizing ideas you have red will assist you in learning whatever topic you choose, and learning new skills engages different types of memory.

Do something you enjoy

Perhaps you enjoy gaming or movies. The fact that I mentioned how technology has the ability to make your memory worse doesn't mean you need to abstain from it completely. A game here and there or a movie a couple of times a week is perfectly all right.

At the same time, if there's a hobby, you're into that doesn't specifically help the brain improve, you're still welcome to do it. Paintball, as an example. Sometimes, you just need to have an afternoon of good, clean fun instead of working towards something. When you do go back to studying, your mind will thank you for it.

Pay Attention

A simple trick to improving memory on a daily basis is simply paying more attention to what's around you. Have a look now. What do you see? Pick an object, and try to describe it in as much detail as possible.

I can see a pink blanket with small blue and white hearts on it. It also has pictures of clouds on it. I think they were once white, but they're currently yellowish. It looks soft and a little fluffy. I can't smell it from here. I believe it's made from cotton.

That's the level of detail you want, perhaps even more. This exercise engages your imagination and brings you right to the moment.

Pair Meditation and Visualization

Meditation is a fantastic daily activity, and you only need to do it for five minutes at a time for it to have a positive effect (Lam, 2015). If you have been meditating for a while and feel like you're past the "focusing on breathing stage," you can pair meditation with visualization.

Close your eyes, and begin by focusing on your breath. Once you feel you're in a good flow, turn your focus to something very specific. Perhaps you want to memorize those Italian animal words, and you're working on the cat on the gate. Perhaps you just want to recall some old, pleasant memories.

Forgo the GPS

This is a slightly scary one if you're unfamiliar with the place in which you live. But it is a great way to kick your memory into high gear very quickly—things happen out of necessity!

It may be wise to try this with shorter trips at first and graduate to longer ones when you're comfortable.

Test Yourself Semi-Regularly

All your work is for naught if you don't see some improvement. While simply feeling like your memory is getting stronger may be sufficient for some, others will want to track themselves, which could also be motivational.

Try to keep a Memory Journal where you can record the changes. This way, you can look back and see how far you've come.

Science may prove facts, but there's no substitution for real-life stories. There are thousands of extraordinary case studies out there, but I've selected five that place particular emphasis on memory. Memory is one of the superpowers we have hidden away inside of us, and while these may be special cases, they're all an indication of how much we can achieve if we're open to possibility and delve within ourselves.

www.ingramcontent.com/pod-product-compliance
Lightning Source LLC
Chambersburg PA
CBHW070124230526
45472CB00004B/1416